IMPROVE YOUR PHYSICAL AND EMOTIONAL HEALTH WITH AROMATHERAPY

LEARN THE FUNCTION OF ESSENTIAL OILS FOR THE HOME, DISCOVER THE GREAT ANTI-STRESS BENEFITS OF AROMATHERAPY

Jorge O. Chiesa

Table of Contents

Introduction: Aromatherapy

You've probably heard the term Aromatherapy and wondered what exactly that funny word "aromatherapy" means. It is the use of vegetable oils in their most essential form to promote mental and physical well-being. The use of the word aroma involves the process of inhaling the odors of these oils into your lungs for therapeutic benefit.

If you've ever used a steam massage for coughing, then you've tried aromatherapy, though not in its purest form. In fact, you've probably been using aromatherapy on yourself and your family for many years without realizing it through steam rubs or electric vaporizers.

Vicks or other steam rub brands use eucalyptus or menthol to clean breasts and stuffed noses. Imagine if you used undiluted eucalyptus essential oil, how clear your lungs would feel.

The term aromatherapy is generally new, beginning to be used in the 20th century, but the practice has existed for thousands of years. It is believed that the Chinese were one of the first cultures to use plant odors to promote health through the burning of incense. The ancient Egyptians used distilled cedar oil mixed with cloves, cinnamon, nutmeg and myrrh to embalm the deceased. The Egyptians also used oils to perfume both men and women.

In the 14th century, when the bubonic plague hit thousands of people, aromas were used to protect against this deadly disease. It is even argued that the popular children's song "Ring Around the Roses" refers to aromatherapy. The lines, "a pocket full of bouquets," supposedly refer to keeping the flower in the person's pocket in an attempt to keep the disease away.

Advancing through the following centuries a growth in books about the use of oils in healing grew.

The Greek alchemist Paracelsus used the term "essence" and focused his study on the use of plants for healing purposes.

While the use of essential oils for perfumery continued to grow over the centuries, their use for medicinal purposes declined slightly until around 1928.

It was then that a French chemist named Rene-Maurice Gattefosse accidentally discovered the use of lavender essential oil to heal wounds.

It is said that he burned his forearm and reflexively placed it in the nearest liquid he saw, which was lavender essential oil. He was surprised to discover that the burn healed quickly and left no scar. It was then that he began to use the term aromatherapy and wrote about the powers of essential oils.

Today, many people are trying to get back to nature. People have seen firsthand the dangerous effects of synthetic chemicals and processed drugs.

The use of all natural essential oils for medicinal, cosmetic and therapeutic purposes continues to grow. Many people have found that the results of using aromatherapy are much greater than those of man-made drugs and with far fewer negative side effects.

Aromatherapy can be used alone or in combination with typical medical treatments. For example, you may use aromatherapy to relieve pain after a surgical procedure. You still get the benefit of surgery, but you don't have to take the powerful and often dangerous pain medications that a doctor prescribes.

The safety of essential oils

The essential oils used in aromatherapy are not always easy to find. The Food and Drug Administration does not regulate essential oils, so you, the consumer, will have to carefully read the ingredients of any oil you buy to make sure it is in its purest form.

To get the maximum benefit from aromatherapy, oils should be used in their purest form.

> ➢ **Finding the best essential oils**

Try to avoid synthetic oils. Essential oils are the only way to obtain a therapeutic benefit from aromatherapy. Many different types of oil will not be cheap and cannot be valued in the same way that the distillation process is varied.

Exposure to light decreases the ability of an essential oil to function, so only buy oils that are sold in dark bottles.

The term "oil" is often a misnomer, as many of them are not oily at all. To test how an oil is distilled, try throwing it on a piece of paper to see if it dissolves quickly and doesn't leave an oil stain.

If you have a health store in your area, buy there instead of a perfumery. They're more likely to have real essential oils for sale.

➢ *Use of essential oils*

Essential oils are very potent when not diluted. To make them safe, you must dilute them with a base oil. Ask your local health store what carrier oils are available, as there are many to choose from.

Follow instructions carefully when making any essential oil compound. If a prescription says a drop, use only one drop. Anyone with a nut allergy should also avoid walnut-derived carrier oils.

Oils should be stored out of the reach of children. If accidental ingestion occurs, contact Poison Control immediately. Pregnant women should consult their physician before participating in any type of aromatherapy.

If you plan to use aromatherapy in infants or the elderly, it is recommended that you use smaller amounts of oil in your prescription. Check with your doctor to make sure it is safe for a particular age group.

Some oils can be toxic if swallowed even in small amounts. In general, unless specified for oral use, essential oils should not be ingested.

Essential oils stored in a cool, dry, well-covered place last six to twelve months. It is important to keep as little oxygen as possible in contact with the oils, so it is important to store them in full bottles, reducing the size of the bottle as needed.

Essential oils should never be placed on the skin in their pure form. They can irritate your skin quickly and cause a chain reaction that will make you sensitive to that oil for life.

People with asthma, epilepsy, or other serious illnesses should consult their physician before using aromatherapy.

To avoid an allergic reaction, place a small amount of diluted oil on a patch of your skin. Cover the stain with a bandage and wait a full day to see if irritation occurs. This can prevent a potentially large allergic reaction to essential oils. Essential oils should be kept away from open flames or fire hazards, as they are all flammable. Never use any type of oil near the eyes. Wash hands thoroughly after handling essential oils to avoid contact with eyes or mouth.

Dangerous essential oils

Some essential oils are very dangerous. These oils should not be sold at all, but they can be purchased via the Internet or in shops with a lower reputation.

Others may be safe in some cases, but can be quite dangerous if used in certain circumstances. Before taking an aromatherapy plan, take your time to understand which oils are safe. Keep in mind that the fact that something is totally natural does not necessarily mean that it is not dangerous to your health.

> ❖ Rosemary, common sage, hyssop, and thyme should never be used if you have high blood pressure.
> ❖ Sweet fennel, hyssop, sage and rosemary should be avoided if you have epilepsy.

❖ Diabetics should not use angelica.

❖ Those suffering from hypoglycaemia should stay away from geranium.

❖ People with kidney problems should be careful if they use juniper, sandalwood or coriander.

❖ Prospective mothers should especially avoid juniper, hyssop, sage, mint, lemon, fennel, lemon verbena, rosemary and gaulteria.

❖ Chlorinated sage should not be used while drinking, as it will intensify the effects of alcohol and make it act like a narcotic.

❖ Chamomile and marjoram should not be used while driving because they cause drowsiness.

❖ Some oils may cause allergies, such as citronella, sage, ylang ylang, and verbana oils.

❖ Oils believed to be carcinogenic are squid and sassafras, should be avoided by all.

❖ Methyl salicylate is the active ingredient of aspirin and sweet birch essential oil. If you use aspirin for medicinal purposes, you should avoid it because of the risk of overdose. It should also be kept away from children, as it smells sweet and is equally dangerous for them.

While the above list are oils that can be dangerous in certain situations, there are other oils that should not be used in aromatherapy at all. These oils can be caustic if inhaled and should be avoided at all costs. This is not a complete list, you should investigate any oil you plan to use before you buy it.

Oils not to be used in aromatherapy

- *Almond* - Contains cyanide that even in small amounts can be lethal.
- *Anise* - Skin irritant.

- ***Arnica*** - May cause dizziness and heart irregularities
- ***Bergamot*** - Severe phototoxic sunburn can occur if exposed to sunlight.
- ***Boldo Leaf*** - Produces convulsions even in small amounts.
- ***Calamus*** - Has carcinogenic (cancer-causing) properties and can cause kidney and liver damage.
- ***Camphor*** - Oral ingestion may be toxic.
- ***Cassia*** - Irritating to skin and mucous membranes.
- ***Cinnamon bark*** - Irritating to the skin.
- ***Costus*** - Skin irritant.
- ***Elecampane*** - Classified as a serious skin irritant.
- ***Fennel*** - May cause epileptic episodes.
- ***Horseradish*** - Irritating to eyes, skin, nose and mucous membranes.

- ***Jaborandi Leaf*** - Oral toxin, skin irritant.
- ***Mustard*** - Irritating to skin and mucous membranes.
- ***Origanum*** - Irritating to skin and mucous membranes
- ***Dwarf Pine*** - Skin Irritant.
- ***Brazilian Sassafras*** - Prohibited by the FDA as carcinogenic and can be toxic even in small amounts.
- ***Savin*** - Skin irritant.
- ***Southernwood*** - Toxic to the skin and if taken orally.
- ***Tansy*** - May cause seizures, vomiting, uterine bleeding, and death as a result of organ or respiratory failure.
- ***Cedarea de Cedro Thuja***
- ***Thuja Plicata*** - Could be a neurotoxin.
- ***Wintergreen*** - May be a skin irritant, especially for those with an aspirin sensitivity. The oil itself is poisonous.

- **Wormseed -** Toxic to liver and kidneys, suppresses heart function.
- **Wormwood -** Consumption can cause visual and auditory hallucinations and addiction. It can also cause seizures and be a neurotoxin.

There are some essential oils that are highly toxic and should never be used under any circumstances.

Essential Oils to Avoid Completely

- Mugwart
- Pennyroyal
- Street
- Sage

How to start with aromatherapy?

If you are starting your journey with essential oils and aromatherapy there are some oils that will help you get started. These are some of the easiest to find and versatile essential oils. They are not only used for therapeutic purposes, but can also be used in many other applications.

Some of these include the manufacture of natural cleaning products and gardening. In addition to the oils, you will need some way to get them into your lungs. An aroma diffuser is a good way to do it.

A scent diffuser quickly puts essential oils into the air and spreads them throughout the room, allowing you to get your therapy simply by relaxing and breathing deeply. They come in all different shapes and styles so you can buy one that matches the décor of every room in your home.

Some operate with the use of an open flame, while others operate with electricity. You can even get the aromatherapy diffusers that work in your car.

> ## *Lavender*

Lavender is a non-toxic and non-irritating essential oil. It is extracted by steam distillation from the flowering tips of the lavender plant. Lavender has long been a popular remedy used to soothe upset stomachs. Lavender has calming and revitalizing properties.

Lavender oil should be light to pale yellow in sweet odor with floral and woody hues. Blends well with other floral and citrus essential oils.

As an aromatherapy it has a variety of health benefits. Its pleasant and soothing aroma makes it useful in the treatment of nerves and headaches, anxiety, depression and emotional stress. It also increases mental endurance and calms exhaustion.

Lavender essential oil is often recommended to treat insomnia, as its smell can induce sleep. Massage with lavender oil can remedy all kinds of pain and discomfort, even when it is deep in the joints.

The lavender oil vapor form is used to treat all types of respiratory problems, including colds, flu, chest congestion, whooping cough, sinus congestion, and asthma. Lavender has been used to promote good blood circulation and stimulate the production of gastric fluids for the treatment of stomach diseases.

> ### Tea Tree

Tea Tree Essential Oil is also a non-toxic and non-irritating product, but may cause sensitization in some people. This oil is extracted by steam distillation from the leaves and twigs of the tea tree.

The tea tree has long been used by Aboriginal people in Australia and is named for its use as an herbal tea. The oil should be pale yellow green or water white. Tea Tree blends well with lavender, sage, rosemary and many spice oils.

Tea tree oil is known to be antibacterial, anti-microbial, antiseptic and anti-viral. In short, it can almost be called a cure for everything because it has many properties to protect against diseases and germs. In Australia it is found in almost every home because of these properties.

Tea tree oil can be used as an antibacterial to cure all types of bacterial infections, including wound treatment. As an aromatherapy it can be used to treat coughs, colds, congestion and bronchitis. It can also keep fungal infections at bay and even cure dermatitis and athlete's foot. The tea tree can be used as a stimulant of hormones and circulation and to stimulate the immune system. Tea tree oil can help eliminate toxins by opening pores and promoting sweating that removes uric acid and excess salt and water from your body.

More essential oils...

➤ *Mint*

Peppermint essential oil is non-toxic and when diluted is non-irritating. May cause skin irritation due to the menthol properties it contains and should be used sparingly.

The use of peppermint has been seen in Egyptian tombs since 1000 B.C. It also has a history of use in China and Japan since early times to treat all kinds of health anomalies.

Peppermint essential oil should be pale yellow or greenish in colour. It has a strong mint aroma. Peppermint works well with other peppermint aromas such as eucalyptus, as well as rosemary and lavender.

Peppermint has been studied in the

scientific community and its health benefits have been proven. Because of this, peppermint oil is available in tablet form. It contains many minerals and nutrients such as iron, magnesium, calcium, omega-3 fatty acids and vitamins A and C.

Peppermint is an excellent remedy for respiratory problems and is widely used as an expectorant to eliminate nasal and respiratory congestion. As an aromatherapy it can be used to treat nausea, headaches, depression and stress. It is also known to treat irritable bowel syndrome. As a skin care product, peppermint oil can improve oily skin and replenish opaque skin.

➢ *Chamomile*

Chamomile is a non-toxic and non-irritating product. It is extracted by steam distillation from the blossoming chamomile plant. Chamomile has been used for more than 2000 years in Europe for medicinal purposes. The oil should be a pale blue that turns yellow as it ages. It will have a warm, fruity, sweet smell. Chamomile mixes well with lavender and geranium, as well as sage and jasmine.

Chamomile is well known for its calming properties. So much so that it can be used in aromatherapy to treat nervous disorders, headaches and migraines. It is also used to soothe allergies and asthma. Many women use it to treat premenstrual syndrome or to relieve the baby's teething or colic.

> *Eucalyptus*

Eucalyptus is relatively new to the aromatherapy family, as it has only been used for centuries. It is not an irritant but can be extremely toxic if swallowed.

It is colorless as an essential oil, but has a distinct pine scent. The essential oil comes from the leaves of the evergreen eucalyptus tree that is native to Australia.

As aromatherapy is used to treat respiratory problems such as sinusitis, nasal congestion, sore throat, runny nose, cough, colds and bronchitis. It is able to treat all these ailments because it is antibacterial, antifungal and natural decongestant.

Eucalyptus also has a fresh and refreshing aroma that makes it ideal for treating exhaustion and mental disorders.

Eucalyptus can also be used in the home as an air freshener, in the manufacture of natural soaps, in saunas for its antiseptic properties, and even in mouthwash or toothpaste.

> ### *Geranium*

Geranium has many healing properties, but can cause some sensitization and influence hormonal secretions, so it should not be used by pregnant women. Geranium oil mixes well with citronella, lavender, orange, lemon and jasmine.

If used in aromatherapy, geranium oil is a great astringent. Promotes muscle stretching to prevent skin from hanging loose.

It has antibacterial and antimicrobial properties to help prevent infections of many types.

Essential oil is also known to be a cytophilactic, which means it stimulates cell growth. It can also be used to treat many mental disorders such as depression, anxiety, anger, and pre-menstrual syndrome.

> ### Rosemary

Although rosemary is considered non-toxic and non-irritating when diluted, it should be avoided by epileptics, pregnant women, and those with high blood pressure.

The floral tips of the rosemary plant go through a steam distillation process to form the essential oil. It should be a clear liquid or pale yellow with a strong herbal-mint odor. Rosemary is one of the first plants to be used for both food and medicine. In the Middle Ages it was used to protect against the plague and to expel evil spirits.

When used in aromatherapy, rosemary oil can help increase mental endurance and increase brain activity. It can also treat depression, mental stress, and forgetfulness. When you inhale rosemary you will immediately feel uplifted, which makes it excellent for fatigue relief. It can also clear the airways and relieve sore throats, colds, and coughs.

Around your house, rosemary can be used as an air freshener and bath oil.

➢ *Thyme*

Thyme essential oil is extracted by steam distillation from fresh or partially dried leaves and flowers of the thyme plant. The oil must be red, brown or orange. It has a spicy, spicy smell. Thyme was one of the first plants used in Western herbal treatments, mainly for respiratory and digestive problems.

Thyme is antibacterial, when used in its aromatic form it can prevent the growth of bacteria inside and outside your body. It is able to cure lung, laryngeal, and pharyngeal infections without affecting the rest of your organs, such as prescription cough medicines. Thyme is also known to stimulate memory and treat depression.

Thyme essential oil is used as an insecticide both at home and in the body. It can also help treat bad breath and body odor.

➢ *Lemon*

Lemon essential oil is not toxic, but can cause skin irritation, so it should be used sparingly. Lemon oil is phototoxic, so exposure to sunlight is discouraged. In Spain, lemon is known as a cure that is used for everything from fever to arthritis.

The oil will have a pale greenish-yellow colour which turns brown as it ages. It has a slight citrus scent and blends well with fennel, lavender, sandalwood and chamomile.

Lemon is very popular for cooking and for its fresh aroma. As an aromatherapy can help relieve stress, anxiety and fatigue.

The scent of lemon helps to increase concentration and alertness and provides a general positive sense to those who inhale it. Lemon has also been used in the treatment of coughs and colds and in the treatment of asthma.

The high amount of vitamins in lemon oil make it a boost to the immune system. It can also improve circulation and stimulate white blood cells, further aiding the ability to fight disease. Lemon has also been used as an aid in weight loss.

As a household cleaner, lemon can be used on metal surfaces such as knives to disinfect them. It can also be used in soaps and facial cleansers as it has antiseptic properties.

➢ *Clove*

Clove oil should be used with extreme care. May cause mucous membrane irritation and severe skin irritation. As such, it should only be used in moderation and well diluted.

The sprouts, leaves, stems and stems of the clove plant are distilled with water to extract the essential oil. It should have a pale yellow color with a spicy aroma.

Clove mixes well with sage, Jamaican pepper, lavender and rose. Cloves have been used all over the world for centuries. It can be used to season foods as well as for medicinal benefits. Cloves contain many minerals including calcium, iron, potassium, and vitamins A and C.

Clove has many health benefits, particularly in the form of dental care. It has germicidal properties that help relieve toothaches, gum sores and mouth ulcers. It may also help relieve a sore throat.

Nail is an aphrodisiac that makes it a great stress reliever when used as an aromatherapy. It can also have a stimulating effect and help relieve fatigue. Cloves can also be used to treat headaches, bronchitis, asthma, coughs and colds. Expectant mothers may use cloves to relieve the nausea and vomiting that often occur during pregnancy.

Clove cigarettes have long been a popular alternative to traditional tobacco. At one time it was thought that the addition of cloves could counteract the negative effects of smoking, which has since turned out to be false. The American Cancer Society points out that there is no scientific evidence that nails cure cancer in any way.

The properties of essential oils

The properties of essential oils are what make them so beneficial. While most of them smell good, that's just a by-product of their real benefit. The term essential oil may seem simple, but in reality they are complicated chemical compounds.

The ingredients of essential oils are organic because they consist of a structure of molecules. This structure is made of carbon atoms and bound by hydrogen atoms.

Oxygen, nitrogen and sulphur atoms may also be present in some essential oils. By becoming familiar with the chemical composition of essential oils, you can understand how they can benefit your health. In turn, you'll also be able to understand why some oils are dangerous.

Main chemical products in essential

oils

✓ Monoterpenes with antiseptic and healing properties.

✓ Sesquiterpenes are anti-inflammatory and anti-infective, they also have calming qualities.

✓ Phenols are a stimulant and are best used in small amounts.

✓ Alcohols are antiseptics, antibacterials, antibiotics and antifungals. They also stimulate the immune system.

✓ Ethers are antibacterial, antispasmodic and anti-inflammatory.

✓ Ketones have relaxing and sedative properties. They are also an anticoagulant and can stimulate the immune system.

✓ Aldehydes can also be used as anti-inflammatories and to calm nerves.

✓ Coumarins are anticoagulants and anticoagulants. They can also be used as sedatives.

Home Combinations

Remember that essential oils are very strong, so follow each recipe very carefully. Less is more when treating with essential oils.

> ➤ *Diffuser mixes*

For attention - 1 drop of cypress, 2 drops of cedar, 2 drops of lemon, 1 drop of pine.

To refill - 2 drops fennel, 3 drops juniper, 3 drops lemongrass.

For alert status - 2 drops of eucalyptus, 3 drops of rosemary, 3 drops of mandarin.

For Motivation - 2 drops of Basil, 4 drops of Bergamot, 1 drop of Clove, 2 drops of Ginger.

For lucidity - 2 drops of Bay, 3 drops of

Ginger, 2 drops of Rosemary.

For Calm - 2 drops of Chamomile, 3 drops of Lavender, 2 drops of Marjoram.

For harmony - 2 drops of Benjuí, 2 drops of Rosa, 3 drops of Verbena.

For peace of mind - 4 drops of Bergamot, 2 drops of Salvia Claria, 3 drops of Cypress.

For Calming - 2 drops of incense, 3 drops of Melissa, 2 drops of Patchouli.

To increase socialization - 3 drops of Litsea Cubeba, 3 drops of Rosemary.

To relax - 3 drops of Lavender, 1 drop of Sandalwood.

For the kitchen - 1 drop of basil, 3 drops of lemon, 2 drops of rosemary.

For the bath - 1 drop of basil, 3 drops of lemon, 2 drops of rosemary.

For the bedroom - 2 drops of bergamot, 3 drops of jasmine, 2 drops of

Ylang Ylang.

For the Office - 2 drops of caraway, 3 drops of incense, 2 drops of ginger.

> ## Household Cleaner Recipes

Aerosol Bathroom Air Freshener

Fill a bottle with 500 ml of distilled water and add the following essential oils:

- ✓ 5 drops cinnamon essential oil
- ✓ 5 drops eucalyptus essential oil
- ✓ 5 drops lemon essential oil
- ✓ 5 drops of essential oil of sage
- ✓ 5 drops thyme essential oil
- ✓ 10 drops bergamot essential oil
- ✓ 10 drops of Citronella essential oil
- ✓ 10 drops Lavender Essential Oil
- ✓ 10 drops of Tea Tree Essential Oil

Shake this mixture well before each use. Spray every day to keep your bathroom smelling fresh and clean.

Lavender and Tea Tree Cleaner

- ✓ 1 tablespoon borax
- ✓ 2 tablespoons white vinegar
- ✓ 2 c. hot water
- ✓ 1/4 t. lavender essential oil
- ✓ 3 drops of Tea Tree Essential Oil

Mix all ingredients and stir until dry ingredients dissolve. Pour into a spray bottle for long-term storage and use. Spray as needed on any surface except glass. Rub and rinse with a clean, damp cloth.

Disinfectant Spray

- ✓ 3 drops of Cinnamon Leaf
- ✓ 5 drops of Pine Needle
- ✓ 2 drops of incense
- ✓ 10 drops bergamot
- ✓ 1/8 t. Solar concentrate
- ✓ 30 ounces of water

Combine essential oils with Sunshine Concentrate and water in a 32-ounce spray bottle. Spray and dry the surface.

Disinfects countertops, stoves and tiles.

Microwave Cleaner

- ✓ 1/4 cup baking soda
- ✓ 1 teaspoon vinegar
- ✓ 6 drops lemon essential oil

Directions: Mix ingredients together to make a paste. Apply to the inside of the microwave with a sponge. Rinse and leave door open to dry for 15 minutes.

Wash the glass turntable by hand. This recipe will eliminate odors from food.

Floor cleaner

- ✓ 1/4 cup white vinegar per bucket of water
- ✓ 10 drops lemon oil
- ✓ 4 drops oregano oil

Basic Formula for Wood Cleaning

- ✓ 1/4 cup distilled white vinegar
- ✓ 1/4 cup water
- ✓ 1/2 teaspoon castilla liquid soap
- ✓ 5 drops jojoba or olive oil

Mix the ingredients in a bowl. Saturate a sponge and squeeze out the excess. Wash tired and dirty wood surfaces. The smell of vinegar will soon dissipate. Dry with a soft cloth.

Creamy gentle exfoliator

- ✓ 2 cups baking soda
- ✓ ½ cup castilla liquid soap
- ✓ 4 teaspoons vegetable glycerin (acts as a preservative)
- ✓ 5 drops of antibacterial essential oil such as lavender, tea tree or rosemary.

For exceptionally difficult jobs, sprinkle with vinegar first, then sit down and continue scrubbing.

Conclusion

The use of essential oils can be beneficial to your health. These products in their natural form promote the general well-being of those who use them. Instead of using complicated man-made chemicals, you use products that nature intended.

Not only can you maintain your health, but you can also protect yourself from diseases like colds and the flu by simply inhaling beautiful fragrances in your home, car or office. Using essential oils will improve your health and raise your energy level.

Aromatherapy can even relieve tension and calm nerves. By using these complex organic compounds you can feel better and look better.

In addition to improving the health of

the head and feet, the use of aromatherapy allows you to avoid the use of other dangerous products. When you use nature's recipes to fight everything from diabetes to heart disease, you're free from the side effects of synthetic drugs.

If you still require prescription treatment, you can use aromatherapy in conjunction with them. Be sure to consult your physician before mixing any chemicals or if you are pregnant or have a continuing health condition.

If you are starting your journey into the world of aromatherapy the kit listed here is a great way to get started. It provides you with commonly used oils that can be used in many recipes.

You should take the time to familiarize yourself with oils that can be dangerous, especially when it comes to your health problems or concerns. Remember that no two people are alike, so what is not irritating to another person may not be irritating to you. Simple tests can help you determine if you will be allergic to an oil.

As a beginner in the field of aromatherapy, you should also consider safety precautions and dangerous oils. Some less scrupulous salespeople, especially online, will continue to sell things you shouldn't use in aromatherapy. If you see something that looks suspicious, trust your investigation and avoid it.

Once you experience the benefits of essential oils, you'll wonder how you've lived without them. Soon your home will be free of man-made chemicals to cleanse and treat disease.

Don't underestimate the power of ridding your home of the smell of bleach and strong household cleaners. Imagine what it does to your respiratory system to carry those odors to your lungs. Now think about what it feels like to breathe fresh, healthy air. This is what happens when essential oils are used to keep the home clean. You and your whole family can breathe easier and feel better. All this through the use of essential oils from nature through aromatherapy.

Aromatherapy is for you. Your goal is to benefit your health and well-being. All the tools you need are some high quality, natural oils and some recipes. The most important thing is to know that you don't have to hurt yourself to keep your body and home free of germs, bacteria and negative energy.

Build a beginner's kit and start healing with essential oils. Once you do, your only job is to breathe.

Now yes, I wish you the best in your results, and remember, everything is practical; theory without action is of no use to you.

A big hug, your friend, Jorge!

By the way, when you achieve your

results little by little, I highly recommend you, if you want to learn how to improve your personal and emotional spirituality, my book, on "HOW TO INCREASE YOUR EMOTIONAL AND PERSONAL SPIRITUALITY", is a book that I am sure will help you a lot on your path of "personal, emotional and spiritual growth".

Without further ado, you can find it in the Amazon search engine, like: "How to increase your emotional and personal spirituality" or looking for my name, like: "Jorge O. Chiesa"... Once again I wish you success in your results!